Prima Fundamentals

How to Eat and Exercise Like a Caveman

RON KNESS

ISBN-13: 978-1534601703

ISBN-10: 1534601708

Contents

Introduction

In this day of age, we have come a long way compared to the cavemen that once walked our planet. Technology has completely changed our world (and not always for the better when it comes to health and fitness). It has made it easier for us to harvest and gather crops and kill animals for meat. – just go to the grocery store. It has become so advanced that fruits, vegetables and animal products are being mass produced at a large scale to accommodate a huge population of people.

Cavemen used to have to walk and sprint for days (bodyweight exercise) to feed their family and there certainly wasn't enough food to feed outside their clan, or last for more than a couple of days. While this may seem terrible, this kind of activity kept them fit even when not fully fed.

Now that we have all this technology helping us gather our food it has created a negative impact on our population. We have now become sedentary throughout our days and barely even have to get up to make our own food.

Instead of hunting for some meat, we drive to our local grocery store, or butcher shop. Instead of picking from fruit trees, we pick it up at the store or even have it delivered to our house.

These conveniences, we have created to make our lives easier, have made us motionless, overweight and unhealthy.

In order to combat our now sedentary way of life, we have created gyms that provide a means to fitness but these machines only help us so much. Most of these machines only target specific areas of the body and cause us to do motions our body was not efficiently designed to do.

Instead, we should be focusing on primal fitness using compound exercises with just our bodyweight to get us to ultimate health.

What Is Primal Fitness?

Primal fitness, also called caveman fitness, is a combination of movements that your body was designed to do to help develop full body strength and health. It is also called functional fitness as it develops muscles used for everyday tasks.

In other words, it is the practice of using your body and what nature has given you to remain fit and healthy. Nature can provide an unlimited amount of resistance and endurance in a way that gyms just cannot deliver.

Cavemen needed to be fit in order to get their food and

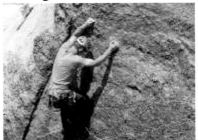

survive out in the wild. These activities probably included walking for miles, sprinting, crawling, swimming and climbing; to name a few. These examples are all great examples of what primal fitness entails.

Now that you do not need to hunt or gather your own food, due to great technological advances, primal fitness can be evolved into a more modern way to mimic these movements.

Primal fitness requires you to use your whole body all at once. Even basic activities that you do to get through your day are a form of primal fitness exercises without you even noticing. Every time you pick up trash or fold your clothes, you are using a wide range of body motions that are the fundamentals of primal fitness.

Just take it one step further by keeping active, with movements that are not repetitive or strenuous to your body throughout your entire day. The key is to keep moving and avoid the black hole of motionlessness.

Basic Primal Fitness Workout Fundamentals

A basic primal fitness workout involves a series of movements that focuses on the whole body rather than targeting one specific range of motion. For example, instead of walking on a treadmill, you should go on a hike.

The key to any primal fitness workout is to move around a lot at a steady pace and to make sure you are using most of your body. Don't over-exercise and have fun. Just avoid being too sedentary throughout your day.

Moving around doesn't have to be a lot of work every time. It's also important to not be repetitive or get stuck on one range of motion to avoid burnout. If hikes start to feel boring, go horseback riding instead.

Examples of modern primal fitness routines:

Squatting: To do a basic squat motion, first stand up straight and move your feet shoulder-width apart. Then lower your body by bending your knees and pushing your hips backwards. Once you can go down as far as you can, stand back up. This motion is used daily when we need to pick up an item or even sit down.

Lunge: A lunging motion was used when cavemen needed to throw their spears. This exercise is done by standing up straight and putting one leg out in front of the other knee.

The back knee is then slowly lowered to the ground. You also do this in your normal daily life when you tie your shoes, for example.

Push: A push motion is any movement where your body weight is pushed away from something. The most popular form of a push exercise is a push-up. To do this you need get down on the ground and put your palms faced down and shoulder-width apart. Then lift up onto your hands and feet with a straight back and your face slightly forward.

To do a full push-up, you must lower yourself down as far as you can go without touching the ground and then push yourself up again. This natural movement is crucial when it comes to survival because your body gains the strength it needs to push your body weight up to walk or move around.

Pull: A pull motion is any movement where a free weight object is being pulled forward or when your body is being pulled toward an object. The most common type of pull motion is a pull-up.

This is done by putting your hands shoulder-width apart on a bar (or tree limb) and then pulling your body towards the object bar and lifting yourself up off the ground. This range of motion is used when you need to pull something, like food, or other larger objects towards you.

Rotation: This is any range of motion that requires your body to twist. To form a basic twist, stand up straight with your feet placed shoulder-width apart. Then twist your upper body left and then right while keeping your hips straight.

Any time you throw an object your body uses a twisting motion. You can do this by playing Frisbee or joining a softball team.

Bend: A bend is when you move your torso down parallel to your hips. Bending is a common motion used when picking up items off the floor to clean the house. You can even exercise in this manner while cleaning by exaggerating your motions.

Gait: This includes walking, jogging, sprinting and jumping. You do at least one of these daily just to live your life.

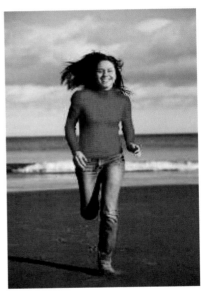

These exercises can be combined to make a highly effective primal fitness workout routine. Just remember these basic motions to be successful.

There is no need for a gym when doing primal fitness. You already have everything you need, provided by nature, to be fit and healthy.

Walking Is a Simple and Powerful Way to Get In Shape

You walk every day. You walk to your car, you walk to your kitchen and maybe you walk your dog. It's as natural as eating or sleeping, and you've probably been walking for a few decades.

So it might surprise you to learn that this fundamental way of moving around is actually quite good for your health and wellbeing.

There are an abundance of mental, physical, and emotional benefits to walking. In fact, walking has been shown to improve sleep, treat depression, and to reverse chronic health conditions like Type 2 diabetes.

10,000 steps and beyond

It takes around ten minutes to walk 1,000 steps. Doctors recommend about 10,000 steps a day, which is the equivalent of about 100 minutes of exercise. Once you've achieved the 10,000 steps a day, you can increase the intensity, steps, and other exercises into your day so that you continue improving your health and fitness.

The great thing about walking

What's uniquely wonderful about walking is that most everyone can do it. You don't need any special skills to walk. Fancy and expensive equipment isn't required. You can be in terrible health or good health and walk.

People all ages and abilities can benefit from walking. You don't even have to go outside to walk. A simple walking treadmill can help you exercise while you work, watch television, or keep an eye on young children.

All at once or in small bites

Walking is also a fitness activity that can be enjoyed on a schedule that fits your needs. For example, if you have time to go for an hour long walk in the morning, great.

If you don't have time for that, you can break your walks up into ten or fifteen minute increments.

Take a short walk in the morning, at lunch, and in the early evening.

Because it's an easy activity to engage in that doesn't require a trip to the gym or specialty equipment, you can fit it into your life more easily. And let's face it - it's a lot easier to talk yourself into taking a walk than it might be to head to the gym.

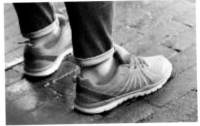

The health benefits will motivate you to start walking...

The mental and emotional benefits will keep you motivated. Walking benefits your mind, body, and emotions. After a week or so, you'll be hooked. Let's start by talking about the amazing health benefits that walking delivers.

Five Benefits of Walking

There are actually dozens of benefits of walking and you'll experience many of them for yourself when you begin your walking for fitness program. However, there are some life-changing benefits that are worth pointing out.

1. Walking reduces your risk for coronary heart disease

You might be surprised to learn that 50% of all deaths in the United States are directly related to heart disease.

It's the single biggest killer. The good news is that regular physical activity, like walking, helps reduce your risk of developing heart disease.

Additionally, it can help you recover from a heart attack or heart surgery and reduce your risk of suffering another heart attack.

2. Walking reduces high blood pressure

High blood pressure has been called the silent killer. When you have high blood pressure, your heart has to work harder to pump blood through your arteries. This causes it to enlarge which then puts you at risk for heart attacks, stroke, and heart failure.

When you walk at a heart-pumping pace, you actually increase blood flow so that your muscle cells get the oxygen that they need. After exercise, your blood pressure will be a bit lower than when you started.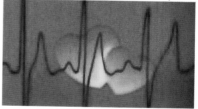

This effect can last for a while. Additionally, walking and exercise help clear up the things that cause high blood pressure, thus reducing your blood pressure and helping to bring it down to more normal levels.

3. Walking improves your blood lipid profile, aka cholesterol

There are two types of cholesterol in your body: HDL (high density lipoprotein) and LDL (low density lipoprotein). They're both needed to build and repair the walls of your cells.

However, too much LDL, which is often called "bad" cholesterol, can raise your risk of heart disease and stroke. In contrast, HDL is often called "good" cholesterol and is also used to help remove fats from your bloodstream. If you don't have enough HDL, you end up with clogged arteries.

Walking and regular exercise help increase HDL and lower LDL. A healthy diet in combination with daily vigorous walking boosts the results.

4. Walking helps you lose weight and keep it off

Obesity is one of the biggest contributors to disease. It causes cancer, heart disease, diabetes and more. And let's face it, extra weight just isn't comfortable. Our lives are too sedentary. We sit too much. Your body was meant to move. And it doesn't have to move in superstar athletic, seemingly superhuman ways.

You don't have to do Cross Fit, ride your bike across the country, or swim the English Channel to get fit. You can walk like you were born to. As you walk, you'll begin to modify your metabolism. You'll burn more calories during the day. You'll also burn calories as you walk.

Walk faster, burn more. Walk longer, burn more. A lifelong walking for fitness program will help you lose weight and keep it off.

5. Walking reduces your risk of Type 2 diabetes

Walking helps you balance your blood sugar by getting your muscles burning the sugars. It increases the number of insulin receptors in your cells which in turn helps move the blood sugar into your cells rather than lingering in your blood and making you insulin resistant.

And if you want to boost the effects, walk after eating. It helps improve blood glucose control and burns more fat and calories.

These are the five most talked about benefits of walking. There are more. Let's take a look at them next because the benefits just keep coming.

Five More Benefits of Walking

When you create a daily walking habit, you're going to be surprised just how much of an impact it has on your life. We're talking about both physical and mental improvements. You'll feel better inside and out. Let's take a look at some of these life-changing benefits of walking.

1. Enhanced mental wellbeing

Exercise reduces stress. It's been proven time and time again through numerous studies. In fact, the National Institute of Mental Health concluded that exercise relieves muscle tension, improves hormone regulation, and has a beneficial impact on how your body responds to stress.

Something as simple as a daily 30-minute walk at a brisk pace can reduce stress-related emotions including anger, depression, tension, sadness, anxiety and more.

Exercise including walking is often prescribed by both physicians and psychiatrists as a way to manage and reduce the effects of stress and depression. For people with moderate depression, daily exercise can significantly reduce symptoms and for those with severe depression, walking and exercise are part of a management plan.

But you don't have to be stressed, depressed, or anxious to benefit from the mental benefits. Walking can induce a state of calm. It helps you feel centered and gives you some perspective on your day and your life.

It gets your heart pumping, which drives oxygen to your tissues including your brain. This in turn helps release endorphins that are known to help create a state of calmness and general wellbeing. If you want to find a way to increase your happiness, try going for a walk every day.

2. More energy and better sleep

Would you like to sleep better? Would you like to have

more energy during the day? Waking can improve both. It can help you have more even energy levels during the daytime and help you sleep better at night.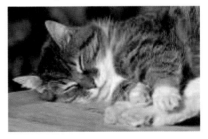

As your heart rate increases, it requires your muscles to use more energy. This in turn has the effect of boosting your metabolism and helping to balance your blood sugar levels. After a brisk walk you'll feel energized for hours as your metabolism continues to hum along.

And because you're requiring your body to perform extra work, it needs to shut down and repair at night. Your mind won't race as you try to fall asleep. Your body's needs will take over and you'll sleep more soundly.

3. Improved sex life

According to a study of women aged 45-55, those that exercised and engaged in a walking for fitness program experienced an increase in libido and improved sexual satisfaction. That's enough to get you in those walking shoes and out the door, right? And bring your husband with you! His libido probably could use a kick in the pants too.

4. Improved self-esteem

A walking for fitness program will help you enjoy life more and feel more positive about yourself. Not only are you taking decisive action to control your life and your health, you'll also start feeling a sense of accomplishment and pride. As your energy improves and you begin to lose weight, your self-esteem will increase too.

5. Improved mobility

When you walk, particularly on uneven surfaces like trails, your body is required to balance and adapt. This helps strengthen your bones, muscles, and tendons and ligaments. The result is improved mobility and a reduced risk of falls as you get older.

You won't have this benefit walking on a treadmill because it's an even surface. However, you still increase your mobility a bit by moving your body and avoiding a sedentary lifestyle.

When you sit and don't move your muscles, they shorten. This reduces your ability to move comfortably. Exercises like walking help restore natural movement.

Okay, so you're motivated to start a walking for fitness program. The benefits are fresh in your mind and you know that it's as easy as putting on your shoes and walking. Let's talk about those shoes next.

While you can walk in anything, including your bare feet, walking shoes can help provide the support and comfort you need to reach your walking for fitness goals.

Choosing the Right Walking Shoe

Having the right equipment when you walk will make your experience the best that it can be. The main piece of equipment that you use for walking is a pair of shoes.

So you want to start your walking program by making sure that you have the right kind for your feet. Your feet aren't formed exactly like anyone else's feet are and you need to cater to the shape of your foot - especially when it comes to the arch.

This can help make a difference in giving you a pleasant walking experience as well as helping you avoid injuries. Even though a pair of shoes might claim to be good to use as walking 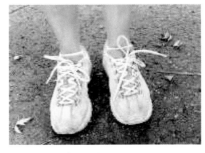 shoes, it doesn't automatically mean that they are.

There are some specific features and details that you'll need to look for. If you're not sure how to choose the right ones, you'll want to follow these tips. One of the most common problems that people run into when they walk is the development of blisters.

Blisters develop when there's friction - something is rubbing an area of the foot. Poor fitting shoes can cause blisters and they can be caused by shoes that are either too loose or too tight.

Shoes that are too loose can rub up and down, such as against the back of the heel. Shoes that are too tight can force your toes into each other and cause pressure blisters.

Wearing the wrong kind of socks can also cause blisters to develop. You'll want to avoid wearing socks that are made of cotton. Cotton socks absorb sweat and moisture, keeping the wetness against your skin.

Choose to wear socks that are made of synthetic fabric instead. These will help keep your skin from staying wet. Something that can also help to keep your feet dry is buying shoes that are lightweight and give you good airflow around the foot.

You'll find this feature if you purchase shoes that are made from lightweight mesh. You do want to be careful that your feet aren't too dry. Dry skin is more prone to the development of blisters than moisturized skin is.

To avoid blisters, you'll want to buy running shoes that fit well, leaving the space of your finger between the end of your toes and the front of the shoe.

Not only can having the right shoes help you keep blisters from forming, but it can also protect you against a common injury with your Achilles tendon.

If you've ever noticed shoes that have the notch at the back, that's what the notch is for. It's called an Achilles notch and it's located at the back center of the shoe.

It's designed that way to offer support to this tendon. You need this support when you're going to be walking - even short distances.

Tearing your Achilles tendon can cause you to be off your feet from a couple of days to a couple of months, depending on the severity of the tear.

Something else that's an important factor to consider with the kind of walking shoes you get is the shock absorption. This is the part of the shoe that's going to be taking the brunt of the impact between your foot and whatever you're walking on.

The surface area where you're going to do your walking will greatly impact your foot's health if you don't have proper shock absorption. Walking on concrete is worse on your feet than walking on dirt or a treadmill.

The more the walking surface gives when your weight comes down on it, the less the strength of the impact. What you want to do is to pay attention to the midsole of the shoe.

This is the area at the rear or heel of the shoe that looks slightly elevated. You want the best cushioning that you can get here. The insole of the shoe is what you also want to check out before buying.

This is the part of the shoe that protects the arch of your foot. If you hold a walking shoe at eye level, you'll see the arch of the shoe. Some people add insoles for extra cushioning, but if you buy a quality shoe, you don't have to do that.

It's important that you buy shoes that are specific toward the type of arch your foot has. There are three types of arches that people have. These are average, high arch or low arch.

Low arches need shoes with more motion control. High arch feet need thicker cushioning. You can tell what kind of arch you have with your feet by wetting the bottom of your foot and stepping onto a piece of cardboard.

For people who have an average shaped arch, there will be a gently sloped indention that resembles the top center of a boomerang arch. If you have a high arch, the imprint of your foot on the cardboard will show only a very small portion of the heel.

The top of the foot imprint may even have a space between it and the bottom of the foot. Low arch feet, also known as flat feet, will show almost all of the footprint on the cardboard.

Those who have normal arches can wear whatever kind of walking shoe that they choose because their feet are better shaped to absorbed shock. High arch shaped feet need a shoe that offers great midsole cushioning, since their arch doesn't give them this necessary support.

Feet with high arches are at a higher risk of joint damage if improper shoes are worn. If you have flat feet, you need to buy walking shoes that offer stability and better midsole support.

Advanced Primal Fitness Workout Fundamentals

An advanced primal fitness workout uses all the range of motions previously outlined above, but used in a way that might not seem like exercise at all. These advanced forms of exercise are the best way to mimic the movements once used so naturally and effortlessly by cave men. That is because those basic body movements are included into actives that are much closer to what they actually did throughout their day.

You don't need to stick to pushups, pull-ups and jumping jacks every day to experience the benefits of primal fitness. In fact these activities are the essence of primal fitness. While doing these activities keep your heart rate at a steady pace. There is no reason to race or over work and risk burning out.

Hiking: Get out on those nature trails and off the paved roads. The hills and nature will provide a natural resistance to your muscles. Start slow, and don't push over your skill level. Once you have built the stamina, find more challenging trails that climb to higher elevations or require you to climb up rocks or trees. You can even take on longer trails that require you to have a backpack for supplies.

Climbing: At work, take the stairs. In nature, learn to climb trees or small rock hills to increase your strength and stamina. For the even more advanced, go rock climbing.

Powerlifting: Power lift objects like tree branches or big rocks. Anything that can be moved in more than in a vertical or horizontal motion is good to try to lift. But, you don't need to do it too repetitively. You could, for example, clear some land of rocks or trees.

HIIT: HIIT stands for "high intensity interval training" and should only be done once a week. This involves doing compound exercises as fast as you can in short bursts of time. For example, doing as many pushups as you can in thirty seconds and then having a short resting period before the next round of pushups or a different exercise to make it circuit training. High intensity interval training helps 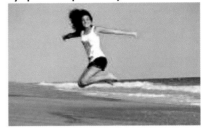 increase your stamina and endurance. Keep these HIIT exercises at a minimum. Primal fitness is about doing things at a relatively good pace and avoids overtraining.

Rest: In the primal fitness world resting doesn't mean to lie around all day. It means to move around less than you did the previous day to insure that your muscles heal properly. Add in a few more hours of rest, but avoid lying around all day. For example, if you went on a strenuous hike yesterday, today you might want to go swimming instead, which works a different set of muscles.

Combining basic and advanced primal fitness workouts is the surest way to see maximum benefits. Keep your exercise at a steady pace and just have fun. Include rest days so your body has time to heal in between high intensity movements.

The advanced primal fitness activities allow you to be healthier in the long run by gradually increasing your strength, stamina and endurance.

Primal Fitness Food Plan

To make the most out of this fitness routine you must combine it with a beneficial and healthy diet. The ease at which we get our food goes contrary to the primal way. So, since you no longer need to work hard to get your food, choose the healthiest food. Eat until satisfied, but not stuffed, and choose food that is closest to its natural form.

The best diet to go with the primal fitness routine is one that was designed on the same principles. The paleo diet is a meal plan specifically made to eat like our primal ancestors once did but in a more modern way. It is said to be the healthiest diet because you were genetically designed to eat this way. To eat paleo simply means to avoid toxins and to eat nutrient-rich foods in their most natural state.

How to Go Paleo

Why would anyone in their right mind want to eat like a caveman? We have wonderfully delicious, lip-smacking foods available on every street corner. Our Paleolithic ancestors did not have this convenience. Sweet, savory, salty delights can be purchased inexpensively, without us having to spend hours in our kitchen.

Our cave dwelling predecessors also didn't have near the choice we have in selecting something to eat.

So why in the world would you choose a Stone Age diet when there are so many eating options available? The answer is simple. The incidence rate of cancer and heart disease has increased dramatically, right alongside the advent of modern agriculture and food processing.

Just because food is convenient, inexpensive or tasty does not mean it is necessarily healthy.

There are chemicals, steroids, artificial flavors, preservatives and unhealthy ingredients added to most processed food. These additions are not made in the name of health. They are made in the name of profits, intentionally forming dangerous addictions to unhealthy food so you keep coming back for more.

Cavemen did not have a McDonald's and Starbucks on every street corner, fortunately for them. They probably didn't even have streets, come to think of it. But you get the point here.

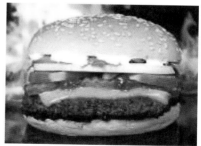

When Paleolithic man needed to eat, he hunted or foraged. He ate natural foods, made healthy by mother nature. He didn't have to worry about additives, refined sugar, salt, preservatives and other chemical nasties ruining his health and well-being.

The reason for returning to a more natural way of approaching your nutritional needs has everything to do with your health.

Human beings are more overweight and obese than ever before. We suffer from more heart disease, cancer and chronic diseases now than at any other time in human history. Nutrition experts, doctors and researchers now understand this is directly tied to the unhealthy processed and fast food diet which so many people unfortunately follow.

What Is The Paleo Diet?

Your ancestors who lived in the Paleolithic era roamed the earth about 15,000 years ago. One of the most important strides humans made at this time was the development of the very first stone tools. Obviously, those human beings had a drastically different diet than the unhealthy Standard American Diet (SAD) eaten by most modern-day societies.

They only ate natural foods.

They ate whatever they could get their hands on, which predominantly meant fish, meat, seeds, vegetables and some occasional fruits. There was no pollution in the air. There were no impurities and garbage being pumped into natural water supplies. The animals and plants during the Paleolithic era were natural products.

They made up the diet of humans, and other carnivores living at that time.

Because of this, your cave dwelling predecessors were extremely healthy, both physically and mentally. Since the way that your body processes foods, and the way it works internally and externally, has not changed significantly since the 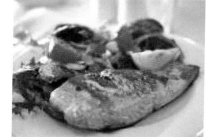 Paleolithic era, adhering to that type of diet can offer you the same wonderful health rewards.

How can your health benefit from a Stone Age dietary approach? Let's take a look.

Health Benefits of a Paleo Lifestyle

Guess what? You may have a much more comfortable living environment then your paleo ancestors did, but they were much healthier than you are. Did you know that high blood pressure, heart diseases, diabetes, high cholesterol and obesity simply did not exist when humans were living in caves 15,000 years ago?

Those difficult, chronic, debilitating and sometimes deadly health conditions are a gift of modern times. This began in Europe when drought forced human beings to start eating wheat. Wheat was combined with water, which became the precursor for what we call bread today.

This eventually led to modern day agriculture and food manufacturing processes. Unfortunately, those food development procedures have led to the creation of refined sugar, simple carbohydrates, trans fats, MSG, table salt, artificial additives and flavors, steroids, preservatives and other unhealthy food ingredients.

Those nutrition nightmares were created so that food could last longer on grocery store shelves. Many of those components, like sugar and salt, are extremely addictive. So human beings end up eating processed food which has much of its nutrients removed, causes unhealthy addictions, and leads to a long list of diseases and illnesses.

A move back to smart eating, enjoying fish, vegetables, meat, nuts, whole foods and some fruits, is what the paleo lifestyle is all about.

The benefits include …

Healthier blood pressure and cholesterol levels.

You will also find that your mental functioning is sharp and clear.

If you have tried to quit smoking before and failed, you will discover, like other paleo converts, that it is easier to give up tobacco on this diet plan.

You will experience plenty of healthy energy, and better sleep patterns.

You also develop stronger, healthier looking skin and hair, and more muscle mass as well.

For those of you who have fought and lost the "Battle of the Bulge" for years, you will also notice immediate and lasting weight loss, helping you regulate a healthy body weight for your size and age (more on that weight loss benefit later).

Why is The Caveman Diet Better Than "Normal" Diets?

One of the most attractive traits of the caveman diet which makes it better than "normal" diets concerns calorie counting. You don't have to do this on the paleo diet. You simply eat foods that are good for you, and eat whenever you are hungry.

When you first adopt a Paleolithic lifestyle, you should track important food metrics, like protein, fat and carbohydrate consumption.

After a few weeks, there will be no need for calorie counting, carbohydrate watching or fat avoidance. This is one of the ways a Stone Age diet is much more attractive than most other diet plans, where daily nutrition tracking is a priority.

Another benefit of this nutrition approach over traditional diets is that it actually works!

This is a lifestyle, not a 30, 60 or 90-day diet. As you probably know, most "diets" may work for a short time, but they are unsustainable. This is 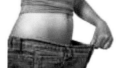 because you do not supply your body with the wonderful nutrients, vitamins and minerals it needs to function properly.

You end up packing on all of the weight that you lost on your miracle grapefruit diet, and in many cases, adding even more weight. On top of that, since you starved your body of the nutrition it so desperately required for the period of time you were dieting, you may have done serious damage to your health.

Another benefit is simplicity.

There are no intricate charts and systems to memorize. You eat healthy, natural whole foods, vegetables, healthy fats, lean meat and some nuts and fruits. That's it. When your nutritional approach is simple, it is much easier to stick to it.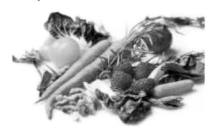

What Is and Isn't Allowed on the Paleo Diet?

Here is where the rubber meets the road. Now we are getting down to brass tacks. (Insert your favorite cliché here if those 2 weren't enough.) What are you allowed to eat on the paleo diet? What is forbidden?

We just mentioned how simple the guidelines of this nutrition approach are. Seriously, get ready to be underwhelmed. The following lists are short and easy to memorize, and illustrate what you can and cannot eat when you want to "pig out" paleo style.

Paleo Rules:

A typical paleo diet has a good ratio of healthy protein, fat, and plant-based carbohydrate and no processed carbs. You should only eat when hungry and avoid portion control. There is no reason to eat if you are not hungry so don't be worried about getting three full meals a day.

A protein should be eaten at every meal, along with a healthy fat and about two servings of low glycemic fruits and vegetables. Eat plenty of organic grass-fed lean meat, seafood, eggs, nuts, seeds, fresh fruit, veggies and a moderate amount of healthy 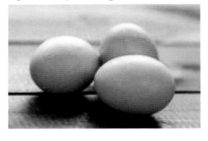 oils like olive, walnut, avocado, coconut and flaxseed.

Drink plenty of water everyday especially when you first wake up, before and after exercising.

It is probably a good idea to supplement vitamin D and probiotics. Other sources of vitamins can be found in fruits and vegetables.

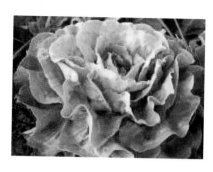

Try to get a different variety of fruits and vegetables each day to get the nutrients and vitamins you need. And, don't forget to get eight hours of sleep each night.

Foods to Avoid:

Grains -- This includes barley, corn, rye, oats and even brown rice.

Legumes -- A legume is the seed or fruit of a plant and is usually enclosed in a pod which includes peanuts, beans and all types of peas.

Oils -- Avoid all processed oils especially hydrogenated oils. Some examples of these oils include margarine, peanut oil, canola oil, and sunflower oil. Even though you can eat some oils, as mentioned above, you should not actually cook with them in large quantities. Eat fats that are in their most natural form as they occur in nature.

Added Sugar - Most items that are packaged or in a can include added sugar such as pasta sauces, soda, fruit and vegetable juices and canned fruits. This is also what is wrong with so-called "fat free" items. During processing, they replace a lot of fat with some type of sugar.

Diary -- This includes all dairy products like milk, cream, cheese and butter. (No, Paleo isn't the same thing as low-carb)

Processed Foods - Most of these foods come in a jar or packages and have added preserves, sugar and are stripped of their nutrients. Common processed foods are chips, cookies, candy, soda, salad dressings, and cereals. Processed foods also include any food prepared at fast food restaurants. A good rule to follow is; "If it's in a box, don't eat it."

Foods To Consume:

Grass Fed Meats – It's important to choose humanely and ethically produced meat that is also lean. Avoid cooking with added fats, sugars, and too much salt. There are plenty of ways you can prepare food without using processed additives.

Fish & Seafood – Look for wild caught fish & seafood and limit it to twice a week. The only reason you need to limit it is due to the fact that there are problems with pollution right now harming the seafood and fish. Source 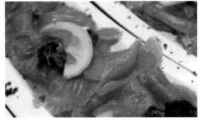 your fish & seafood well and you can eat more.

Fresh Fruit – Choose more berries and fruits that are lower on the glycemic level when you eat fruit, and limit it to two or three servings a day. If you were to look at your plate, $1/4^{th}$ of your plate should be fruit.

Fresh Veggies – About 1/2 of your plate should consist of lightly steamed fresh vegetables without any additives. Choose real veggies and not grains. Corn is a grain, not a veggie. Lima beans, are well – beans. Choose broccoli, cauliflower, spinach, Brussels sprouts and more.

Eggs – You can safely eat up to three eggs per day, and what's more, they are good for you. They're rich in omega fatty acids and B12.

Nuts & Seeds – Choose raw, not roasted nuts and seeds. Nuts can cause weight gain in some people so limit them to one or two handfuls per day. If you need to lose weight and are having issues, stop eating the nuts and eat seeds instead.

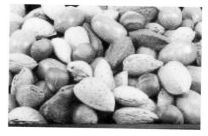

Healthy Oils – Limit oils but you can use coconut oil in recipes, olive oil, and of course eat an entire avocado each day if you like.

That's it. That is how simple it is to adhere to a healthy, beneficial caveman diet plan that makes you look and feel great.

What Fats Can I Eat on the Paleo Diet?

Get ready for a real shocker! Fats are a big part of the paleo approach to living a healthy life. Yep, fat can be a good thing.

Your body needs either carbohydrates or fats to produce energy. If it has neither of these, it will begin to eat up your muscle mass to develop energy. Obviously, you don't want that.

So since you are extremely limiting your carbohydrates, which is a big factor leading to the health benefits of the paleo diet, you need to produce energy from some other source.

That is where healthy fats come in.

Not all fats are created equal. Some fats are good for you, others are not. Accordingly, you are probably wondering what fats you should be eating more of as a part of the paleo diet.

Below we have listed some healthy and not healthy fats, those which are and are not approved as a part of the caveman diet.

Healthy Fats (Paleo Approved)

- Omega-3 fatty acids

- Coconut oil

- Butter

- Ghee

- Animal fats

- Extra-virgin olive oil

- Avocado oil and avocados

- Lard

- Palm Oil

Unhealthy Fats (Paleo Denied)

- Canola

- Corn

- Vegetable

- Soybean

- Safflower

- Sunflower

- Cottonseed

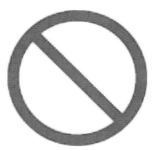

Those "bad" fats are polyunsaturates. Over-consumption can lead to high blood pressure, a depressed immune system, cancer, obesity, diabetes, sterility and inflammation.

Is Dairy Paleo?

As you can see from the unapproved foods mentioned earlier, dairy products are included. Strict paleo practitioners absolutely avoid dairy products. Other paleo lifestyle adherents eat dairy sparingly. So what's the deal? Can you eat dairy, or not, as a part of the caveman diet?

Honestly, it depends on who you talk to. Some caveman dieters say if you can locate high-fat, raw, natural dairy products, then dairy is acceptable. Others point out that cave dwelling humans didn't eat cheese and drink milk, so dairy is definitely out.

You have to make the decision for yourself.

Strictly, dairy is forbidden. When you take a look at 99.9% of the dairy products you find at your local grocer's, you will see they are definitely on the no-no list. Processed goods are not allowed on the paleo diet. Most cheese, milk and other dairy products are heavily processed, so they have no place in this healthy nutrition approach.

However, as mentioned above, if you can find raw, organic, natural dairy products, you have to make the decision for yourself if you are going to include this usually restricted food item in your paleo practice.

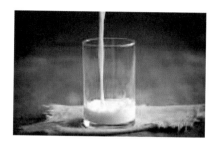

Are Grains and Legumes Paleo?

The unapproved paleo food list includes cereal grains and legumes. Your Paleolithic ancestors ate whole foods that included meat and plants, but industrialized plants such as wheat and other grains were not available. Grains are also very carbohydrate-rich.

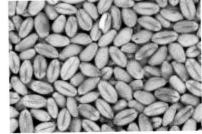

This can cause a drastic spike in blood sugar levels, which can in turn lead to obesity and eventually diabetes. Phytates, gluten and other "anti-nutrients" are often found in grain products as well. For this and other reasons, grains should be avoided on the paleo diet.

As far as legumes are concerned, they simply were not a part of your ancestors Stone Age diet. Only a few Paleolithic people ate legumes, the Australian Aborigines and some Kalahari Desert tribesmen. Additionally, they often contain toxic ingredients like phytic acid and lectin.

The basic premise of the paleo diet is to get back to the healthy approach to nutrition our ancestors enjoyed. That means steering clear of foods which they did not eat. Our Paleolithic brethren were very healthy. As noted, things like heart disease and cancer simply didn't exist back then.

This is because our ancestors ate a very healthy, all natural diet. They ate very few carbohydrates, and more fats. This caused their bodies to burn fat for fuel, which made them lean and healthy.

Avoiding grains and legumes is a part of that approach.

In the end, the choice is up to you. Probably enjoying a few grains, beans or peanuts here and there may not have a drastic, negative health effect. However, it could start you on the slippery slope to straying outside the boundaries of a paleo diet.

Why (and How) the Paleo Diet Works for Health and Weight Loss

If you have a weight problem, you probably have a carbohydrate problem. Carbohydrates and other simple starches can be effectively used for energy sources. However, when you take in too many carbohydrates, those excess carbs tend to get stored as fat.

The paleo diet naturally restricts the amount of carbohydrates you ingest to a healthy level. Your blood sugar doesn't spike, you don't run the elevated risk of developing diabetes which too many simple carbohydrates in your diet can deliver, and your body burns fat for energy.

This process is what kept your Paleolithic ancestors lean, strong and healthy. It also leads to all day energy stores. Since fat is your energy fuel, and you consume a limited number of carbohydrates, you don't develop excess body weight.

Modern-day health professionals agree that overweight and obesity are severe health problems. When you start carrying around too much weight, your cardiovascular, respiratory, skeletal and digestive systems have to work much harder. This can lead to a long list of health problems.

Limiting carbohydrates and eating natural, nutritious foods allows your body to properly regulate itself. All of your internal and external processes and body parts function as they should.

You don't have to attempt to look great, feel great and enjoy the best health of your life ... it just comes naturally as a byproduct of eating a smart, healthy, natural diet and avoiding modern-day processed and unhealthy foods.

How to Transition to a Paleo Diet

There are certain tips that make transitioning to a paleo diet easier. We highlight a few of those in this section. You should also consider whether you are going to take the paleo plunge all at once, or parcel it out over time. You know yourself better than anyone else.

Either you are going to be successful slowly moving to a paleo lifestyle, or your chances of success are better when you make an immediate and total switch. Whether you decide to transition slowly or quickly to a caveman diet, the information contained in this section will improve your odds of making this substantial nutritional change with as few hiccups as possible.

Go Paleo Overnight or Transition Slowly?

There are arguments to be made for slowly moving to a Paleolithic approach for nutrition. Some would argue that an all-or-nothing, overnight change makes more sense. If you are sold on the health benefits of a Stone Age approach to eating, and you don't know if you should make a wholesale change overnight, or transition gradually, keep the following points in mind.

Gradually Learning to Eat Like a Caveman

Are you the type of person who likes to "test the waters" before diving into the pool? If so, you will probably decide to take the same gradual approach to your paleo transition.

Here are a few pointers to help you make the move slowly, but successfully.

Write down 3 or 4 of your favorite foods that you are going to have to sacrifice. Replace one of them each week over the next month, rather than depriving yourself totally right away. You should also make a list of all of the non-paleo foods in your home.

Box up and donate those foods which you know you will not have a problem doing without. Then take a look at the remainder of your list. These are the foods you should gradually replace over the next 30 days. Creating a food replacement journal and planning for the removal and addition of specific foods on a daily basis will improve your odds for success.

People often think of the willpower issue of drastically changing your dietary approach. The mental difficulties associated with this change can be significant. However, there are also physical side effects which sometimes accompany a move to the Stone Age diet which make a slow and gradual transition sensible.

Constipation and an upset stomach are 2 issues that paleo diet newbies sometimes report. Your body is going through a pretty substantial change. A withdrawal known as the "Carb Flu" is often experienced when someone begins eating drastically fewer carbohydrates than they were used to.

If you feel run down, have little energy, are irritable and "out of it" like when you have the flu, these are typical carb flu symptoms. They usually pass in a few days.

As you enter ketosis, your body begins to burn primarily fat instead of carbs for energy. Unfortunately, this can lead to what is known as "Ketogenic Breath". The result is a mildly unpleasant aroma to your breath, which can be defeated by chewing on cilantro or mint.

This side effect does not affect everyone.

You also may experience hypothyroidism. This is when your thyroid slows down, which is what leads to the fatigue, sluggishness and low energy the carb flu is symptom eyes by eat more paleo friendly vegetables to keep your carbohydrate level where it needs to be.

Finally, you are going to have serious carb cravings. An extra-large order of French fries or a couple of bags of potato chips will seem like absolute heaven. Don't worry, these cravings pass after a week or two.

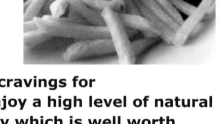

The good news is, when you no longer experience cravings for carbohydrates, you will enjoy a high level of natural energy and a mental clarity which is well worth waiting for.

From Processed and Fast Foods to Paleo and Healthy Fats Overnight

Some people prefer quick change. They decide on a plan of action, and they get started right away. As opposed to a gradual paleo transition, this may be what you are planning on.

Performing an "overnight" paleo change is also a good idea if your willpower is weak. This removes any and every non-paleo food temptation from your home all at once. You are basically forcing yourself to begin adhering to the caveman diet with an "all in" approach.

This doesn't require extensive planning as with a gradual transition. Study your paleo foods list. Do some reconnaissance shopping at your local supermarkets and grocery stores.

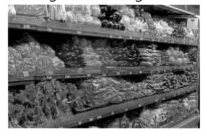

Make a meals list for your first 2 weeks or 30 days. If you are fortunate enough to be making this move with a partner, one of you can be cleaning out your pantry, refrigerator and freezer while the other is shopping for paleo approved foods.

Paleo Nutrition Tips

Anytime your body is subjected to massive change, mental and physical issues can arise. We discussed that earlier, when you decided whether you wanted to ease into a healthy paleo lifestyle, or make a sudden and lasting change.

There are also other considerations which need to be mentioned. The following tips, reminders, pointers and information will help you successfully move from the SAD eating habits you currently have, adopting and benefiting from a Stone Age diet plan.

Make Sure You Are Eating Enough

Going paleo means you're going to be eating a lot of foods which are full of healthy dietary fiber. These foods are also nutritionally very rich, and extremely good for you. This combination means that you can quickly feel full.

That may not sound like a problem. However, some people transitioning from a predominantly processed food diet to a Paleolithic lifestyle initially do not consume enough calories. This is because many of the fiber-rich vegetables you will be eating do not have near the calorie load of the nutritionally nightmarish food you are used to.

For instance, one cup of broccoli delivers just 55 cal. and 6 g of carbohydrates, but delivers more than 2 dozen essential nutrients. That single cup of broccoli fills you with a full 21% of the fiber you need in an entire day.

A cup of fast food French fries delivers between 200 and 300 cal. and a whopping 30 g of carbohydrates.

So when you eat broccoli, and other paleo friendly foods, you may feel full before you have eaten a healthy number of calories on the day. This filling, nutritious aspect of the caveman diet is why it is so great for helping you regulate a healthy body weight. You should still, however, track your calorie intake daily, and make sure you are not starving yourself calorie-wise.

You should also have target numbers for daily carbohydrate consumption as well. Paleo nutrition trackers are available as free downloads for most smart phones and computers. They provide a perfect way to ensure you are getting the correct amounts of calories, carbohydrates and healthy fats in your daily paleo diet plan.

One of the wonderful benefits of the paleo plan is not having to track and count calories. At the beginning, using a paleo nutrition tracker will help you figure out how much of what food you need to be eating each day. After a while knowing what to eat every day will become second nature, and you may not need to refer to a nutrition tracker.

Understand How to Build a Balanced Paleo Plate

Eating should always include a plan. That plan should account for the right amounts of fats, carbohydrates and protein for each meal. With a Paleolithic lifestyle, aim for the following serving sizes at each meal.

Eat about a thumb sized amount of fat at each meal. This is roughly 1/4 to 1/2 of a small avocado, or 2 to 3 tablespoons of nuts. If you add oil or fat to your meal, this is the equivalent of 2 or 3 teaspoons.

You should eat at least, but not much more than, protein equivalent to the size of 1 or 2 of your palms. Your body can only process so much protein at the time, so eating more than that is wasteful.

Include a fistful of carbohydrates at each meal.

Fill the rest of your plate with vegetables.

Herbs and spices approved on the paleo plan can be used liberally, as they are extremely healthy, and virtually absent of calories, carbohydrates, protein and fat.

Eating Paleo Away from Home

Sometimes you want to enjoy a meal out. This means dining at the home of a friend or a restaurant, without wrecking your paleo nutrition plans. At a restaurant this can simply be accomplished by speaking with your server, chef or a member of the restaurant management staff.

Ask them exactly how their food is prepared. Mention that you practice of paleo lifestyle and give them a quick and simple definition if need be. The key is asking a lot of questions, and realizing that eating away from home does not give you the wide variety of paleo choices you enjoy in your own kitchen.

Another great tip is to eat before you head out. Do some shopping around, and talk with your Paleo-minded friends.

Once you find a restaurant that gives you plenty of choice while also adhering to your dietary constraints, convince your friends and family members to meet you there for dinner.

You should also probably totally avoid restaurants which specialize in pizzas and sandwiches. There just aren't going to be any reasonable alternatives that fit your lifestyle.

Why not tell your waiter or waitress you have a gluten allergy? Ask if whatever you are considering ordered is breaded. Ask if they are capable of using olive oil instead of their standard cooking oil.

Batch Cooking the Paleo Way

Batch cooking makes sense no matter what type of dietary approach you take. You take the time to cook once, making all of your meals for the following week. Website Paleo.com recommends keeping a weekly meal planner. They also suggest cooking on the same day every week. On the day you are going to batch cook, pull out your meal planner. This is when you keep information like when you are cooking for friends, how many meals are required for how many people each week, and other mealtime specifics.

After you plan what meals you're going to eat in the following week, take your meal planner to the grocery store, using it as a shopping guide.

Back at home, focus on one pot recipes like casseroles, soups and stews. These can be made in large batches, and portioned off. You can also use the batch approach to vegetables and meats, cooking in large quantity and then freezing and refrigerating individual serving sizes.

Simple Paleo Meal Ideas

Veggie Omelets: Whip three eggs with a fork until blended well; add a couple tablespoons of water to make them fluffier. Using a non-stick pan and a little coconut oil to coat the pan, heat the skillet until hot. Pour in the eggs. Let cook for a while, and then flip over. Now add fresh veggies like onions, bell peppers, broccoli, and even mushrooms until heated through. If you prefer your veggies well cooked, cook them before adding the egg mixture.

Smoothies: Smoothies are super simple to make and can be made to your tastes. While smoothies were not made in the wild, food was more nutritious before modern farming practices messed up the vitamins in the food. In a high speed blender put some cashews that have been soaked in filtered water for 1 hour and drained. Add a banana, 1/4 an avocado, 1/4 cup of ice, 1 cup of black coffee, chilled, and blend well.

Oven-Roasted Vegetables: This is probably the easiest meal, along with roasted skewers, you could ever make. Simply pick your favorite vegetables and cut them making sure each vegetable is relevantly the same size. Coat with a few tablespoons of coconut oil and sprinkle some seasonings over the top. Cook in the oven for about 40 minutes or until soft in a 400-degree oven. Vegetables that are perfect for this include sweet potatoes, zucchini, Brussels sprouts, bell peppers, onions, and squash.

Roasted Skewers: You can make skewers with any animal protein and fish you can think of added with fruits and vegetables. Take a few cubed pieces of steak, chicken and shrimp and push it through a skewer. Cook on a grill or a grill pan until it's evenly cooked. To make sure all the meat is cooked evenly only put one type of meat or fish on each skewer. Another great combination is chicken and pineapple or shrimp with lemon garlic sauce. A lemon and garlic sauce can easily be made with a few cloves of garlic, a squeeze of lemon, and a couple tablespoons of coconut oil.

Pre workout paleo meal ideas:

Small chicken salad: Mix together 4 ounces of grilled chicken, about a handful of kale, one fourth of an avocado and one apple diced. Make a quick vinaigrette with olive oil, lemon juice and pepper.

Smoothie: A small green smoothie that includes a handful or two of spinach, one banana and sweetener such as honey blended with a good amount of water.

Nuts & Seeds: A small handful of nuts like almonds or seeds like sunflower.

Post workout paleo meal ideas:

Throw about two bunches of spinach and or kale in a saucepan with a few tablespoons of water. Cook until all the kale is tender and the water is evaporated, for even more flavor you can use broth. In a bowl whisk about 3 eggs and add it to the saucepan with the spinach. Add some seasonings, garlic and other vegetables of your choice. Spread it evenly across the sauce pan and cook until it's about half way done and then throw in a 400-degree oven for about ten to fifteen minutes.

Another quick idea is a baked sweet potato or one or two small bananas. Combining a paleo diet with a primal fitness routine can amp up the health benefits of both. The great thing about being natural and eating natural food in the right amount for your body is that you will lose weight if you need to. You'll also have an increased amount of energy, clearer skin and lift that dreaded mind fog.

It's important to let your body be the guide to how much you eat. If you pay attention you will be able to differentiate between hunger and thirst and only eat when you are hungry and stop eating just as you get full (not stuffed). Each meal should include a ratio of about 1/2 veggies, 1/4 protein, and 1/4 low glycemic fruit.

How Does Primal Fitness Differ From CrossFit?

CrossFit is a fitness program designed to increase overall body health and strength. It involves functional movements that are constantly varied and performed at high intensity during a specific time frame. The idea behind CrossFit is to allow someone to become an athlete in every category in a short amount of time.

CrossFit is typically a class that involves a variety of exercises that is slightly different every day. They have elements from several different categories including high intensity interval training, Olympic weightlifting, plyometrics, powerlifting; gymnastics and it even includes movements and techniques from many other sports.

Although CrossFit and primal fitness both focus on developing overall body strength by using natural movements the idea behind each are completely different. Here are a few ways CrossFit is different from primal fitness.

CrossFit is Class Oriented -- To get the best benefits from CrossFit, you need to join a class. This fitness program thrives on a community. This is to make sure you get the most variety from your workouts and to help you set times for each workout.

CrossFit Always Involves High Intensity Workouts -- Primal Fitness involves some high intensity workouts but the goal is only about once a day. Every workout for CrossFit is meant to be performed at a high intensity.

CrossFit Periodically Measures Your Fitness -- Primal fitness and CrossFit both have the goal to create overall body fitness but they measure it in a completely different way. CrossFit will periodically have benchmarks to count how many times you can do a specific exercise in an allotted amount of time to measure your fitness.

Primal does not have a specific measure of fitness because it's more about being natural. You will notice your level of fitness as you go up because you will be adding in more movement with each passing day.

CrossFit Is a Brand -- CrossFit was developed by Greg Glassman who wanted to create a brand to promote overall fitness.

The overall main difference is that primal fitness is about getting moving and living the life as hunter/gathers once did, but in a more modern world. Instead of going to one class each day, you can do primal fitness all day long without being burned out.

Primal fitness is a way of life. It's to help you escape a motionlessness life and be more active throughout your entire day. It is not about vanity and determining how fit you really are. It's simply being active and healthy without overtraining.

Primal Fitness vs Standard Gym Workout

The great thing about primal fitness is that you get to ditch the gym. In a gym, it's boring, repetitive and eventually your results will be at a standstill. Also, most of the machines at the gym can lead to serious injury and might not even produce results.

Of course, getting any kind of exercise is a good thing because it gets you active and prevents heart disease. But, some fitness routines, like primal fitness, have far more benefits than what is provided by machines at the gym.

Gyms Are Boring & Expensive

Let's face it, the gym is not the most exciting place to go and most people want to avoid it for many reasons. It can be pricy, overcrowded and small. Not to mention, smelly.

The moment you get the courage up to go, the one machine you wanted to use has been taken. Then, to make your trip worth it you try out other machines. These machines often do not have the best directions and using them wrong can cause serious harm to your body.

Gyms Can be Overwhelming

It can even be quite overwhelming when you are just starting out with your new health routine and actually need to lose a few pounds. Gyms often have poorly trained and paid personnel who don't really know much about health or fitness.

With primal exercise and activities, you can avoid all this and get even better benefits.

You Can be Injured & Results are Limited

Most exercise machines only target specific areas of the body. More times than not, people tend to stick to the machines they know how to use. This causes them to only work out a few areas of the body every time they go.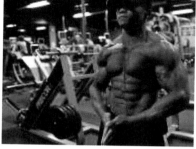

This means their results are very limited. The results they get could be taken a bit farther if they add in some primal exercises that require the whole body such as <u>burpees</u>. These exercise really workout your whole body because it requires you to use your own body weight to complete it.

Gyms Can Make Movement Feel Negative

When you end up dreading to go to a place it oftentimes ends up feeling like a chore. When something becomes a chore people, more times than not, decide to avoid it. Then they are in the awful routine of saying "I'll start tomorrow" or "I really need to start my fitness routine again."

People easily find themselves in this awful pattern because they believe that the gym is the only place they can get the best results. This is simply not true. Getting out in your environment provides unlimited results and benefits.

You can avoid this awful routine by finding an activity that doesn't seem like a chore. Something that'll make you excited to get out and do it. Primal fitness can be really fun if you find the right kind of activity for yourself and because primal fitness has so much to offer, you can be sure you will find something you'll enjoy.

And before you know it, you will have the results you want and need. You will be happy and stress free knowing you are doing the right thing.

How to Get Started with Primal Fitness

Now that you understand what primal fitness is all about, it's time to jump in and get moving every single day. It really is that easy.

The goal of primal fitness is to make sure you are not stuck in bad motionless habits that the culture has seemingly fallen into. There are so many ways you can get yourself moving throughout the day that can be fun and rewarding.

Here are a few steps you should follow to get started with primal fitness:

Always keep moving: This is the easiest thing you can do. Instead of sitting and watching TV or playing on the computer, just get up and start moving around. Clean your house, go for a walk, and dance around your house. Anything that moves your body will work. The key to primal fitness is to mimic the lives of the hunter/gather.

In primal times people were consistently in motion. They did not have computers or television to sit in front of for hours on end to entertain them. Their whole day consisted of getting food to survive. Eventually, you will want to make sure that the time you are moving around outweighs the time you are sitting around.

Slow and steady: Don't be overwhelmed and think you need to start climbing trees or walk around your neighborhood for a couple of miles right away. Start out slow and steady. Figure out what your day-to-day schedule is like and fine ways to incorporate a few exercises. Then plan for a little walk before dinner.

Gradually add in more exercises as time goes on and when you start feeling a little more comfortable.

Develop a routine: You will want to create a seven-day fitness plan that is tailored to your interests. Find all body workouts you enjoy doing and plan to do them every day. Include a rest day and a day where you do some high intensity interval training. HIIT should be the hardest day of the week.

Try something new: Once a week explore new activities. This is a great way to figure out what you really enjoy doing. This way you can easily get moving without feeling like it's a chore. Take a dance class such as ballroom dancing, or line dancing. Incorporate movement into your life by doing simple daily chores to keep your home and environment clean.

You might seem a little overwhelmed at first, but if you follow those steps you will quickly realize how easy it is. You are probably thinking primal fitness is too much work and there is no way you can ever incorporate that much exercise. But, the benefits you will receive will be worth it. You are going to be so energized and happy that you won't want to stop.

Before you know it your television and Internet time will be cut in half and your days will be much more productive. (Tip: When watching TV use that time to exercise, do some planks or lunges.)

Three Benefits of Primal Fitness

Primal fitness has many health benefits because it's a fitness routine that will be engrained to your everyday life. If you are active more than you are sedentary benefits are going to make their way to you. Below are only a few of the many benefits you will receive on this lifestyle fitness plan.

Overall Health – Due to the amount and variety of exercise, activities and food, you will develop overall strength and health. Your strength will increase throughout your whole body. The more you move and avoid being sedentary, the more your energy will increase.

Avoiding the couch, computer desk, and too much sitting and getting out in nature will increase your flexibility and make it easier for you to be mobile. Flexibility and mobility are increased because with primal fitness you are encouraged to do workouts that focus equally on all muscle groups.

Increased Happiness -- In order to imitate what prehistoric humans did, you have to get outside in nature. Nature is where all the exercise and moving should take place. Because you will be outside you will be exposed to more sunlight and vitamin D. Sunlight has been proven to increase happiness. So many people are suffering from vitamin D deficiencies today due to being stuck indoors too much.

Even without sunshine, exercise gets endorphins moving which make you feel good and lowers incidences of depression. Increased happiness leads to many other health benefits as well. Such as lower blood pressure, less stress, more energy and a better functioning immune system. Happiness is even associated with a lower risk of cardiovascular disease.

Weight Maintenance or Loss -- If you combine this fitness lifestyle with a whole foods diet, you'll be able to lose extra weight if you need to, and maintain once you've reached your goal. The best diet to pair primal fitness with is a whole foods diet such as the paleo diet.

That is because the paleo diet is said to be similar to what hunters and gathers once ate. Not only would you be exercising similar to what earlier humans once did, you would also be eating like them which are the ingredients for success.

Primal fitness is a workout routine that is meant to emulate the physical activity earlier humans once did. To survive, early man had to hunt and gather their food and even run and fight against predators. They also did not have the modern conveniences that we do now with technology and instant (fast) food.

Now that we no longer need to hunt and gather our food or fight against predators, we have become sick, overweight and unhealthy. Primal fitness was designed to combat disease, obesity and to get you back to your primal or natural state.

Get Started Today!

All primal fitness exercises are natural movement that your body is designed to perform, moving the entire body. These basic movements include squatting, lunge, pushing, pulling, rotation, bend and gait.

The motions can be used to make more advanced primal workouts or you can simply focus on being busier each day so that you move around more than you sit doing the normal things you need to live your life such as cleaning, yardwork, playing with your children and walking and enjoying nature.

The advanced workouts can include longer and more progressive hiking, rock climbing, and some high intensity training, such as running sprints while walking, or dropping and doing as many pushups as you can do. You can also include powerlifting using items you already have around the house.

The main focus of primal fitness is to get moving at a slow and steady pace and avoid overtraining by incorporating days of less movement after days of strenuous movement.

To get the most results of a primal fitness exercise routine, eat a whole foods diet like the paleo diet. This diet is rich in proteins, vegetables, fruits and also includes raw nuts and seeds. When eating a paleo diet you should avoid added sugars, processed foods, sugar, hydrogenated oils, grains, legumes and dairy.

As long as you avoid any items that are in a can or package you should do just fine. When shopping stick to the outside of the grocery store where all the fresh food is avoiding the inner isles where the packaged food lurks.

To successfully mimic ancestral fitness, you need to get outside and ditch the gym. Gyms are overpriced, uninteresting and monotonous. They also encourage a bad habit of laziness because they can be overwhelming and overcrowded.

Not to mention if you do manage to get to the gym, you may think that now it's okay to sit around for four hours playing on Facebook, or binge watching **Orange Is The New Black**. Not to mention that most gym machines only target specific muscles in the body unlike primal fitness which encourages overall body strength.

Thankfully, getting started is easier than you think. You already have all the components needed to get started. Start by looking at your daily schedule and gradually add in more exercises. Continue by adding more interesting and more advanced movements with each passing week, month and year.

Find activities that you find fun and do them. But, also remember the normal daily activities that you need to do to keep a clean, healthy home environment like housework, yardwork, and even laundry.

It's amazing what a workout some of those activities can be if you just exaggerate the movements and do them more often.

Other Senior Health and Fitness Books by This Author

If you would like to read more about Senior Health and Fitness, here is a list of the <u>titles, CreateSpace links and descriptions:</u>

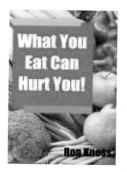

What You Eat Can Hurt You

https://www.createspace.com/4963196

Do you know that certain foods increase your risk for inflammation, disease and illness? It's true! And certain foods can help cure and heal you if you do get sick. Knowing which foods to eat and which ones to avoid empowers you to manage your own health.

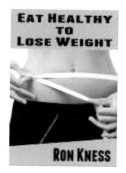

Eat Healthy to Lose Weight

https://www.createspace.com/4962939

As you read through our book, we show you which foods you should and should not be eating to reach your weight loss goal, along with discussing how to maintain your weight loss and stay within a few pounds of your goal weight. Banish the weight you keep gaining back each time by learning how to live a healthy lifestyle.

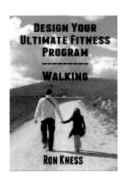

Design Your Ultimate Fitness Program - Walking

https://www.createspace.com/5252272

In my book Design Your Ultimate Fitness Program – Walking, we discuss the considerations that need to be made when designing a custom walking program, along with:
• Equipment needed
• Wearable technology you can use to track your walking
• And how to make walking more challenging

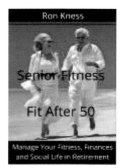

Senior Fitness – Fit After 50: Learn How to Manage Your Fitness, Finances and Social Life in Retirement

https://www.createspace.com/5474751

Inside you will discover answers to your most pressing questions:
• What do I need to know about downsizing my home?
• What are the best tips for staying healthy as you approach your 50's?
• When should I start planning for retirement?
• I am worried about being lonely once I retire, do others feel the same?
• Is it worthwhile to carry two homes during retirement? And more...

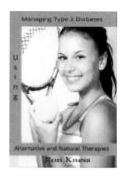

Managing Type 2 Diabetes Using Alternative And Natural Therapies

https://www.createspace.com/5401244

While Type 2 diabetes can be managed medically, there are many alternative natural and holistic methods of therapy and treatment that can further enhance quality of life and minimize the effects of this disease. In this book, I discuss 12 different types, including yoga, reflexology and acupuncture to name just three.

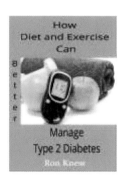

How Diet and Exercise Can Better Manage Type 2 Diabetes

https://www.createspace.com/5404845

Of the different types of diabetes, only Type 2 can be reversed. In my book How Diet and Exercise Can Better Manage Type 2 Diabetes, we reveal the three things you can do to best manage your disease, including:
• Diet
• Exercise
• Weight management

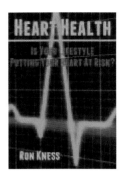

Heart Health: Is Your Lifestyle Putting Your Heart at Risk?

https://www.createspace.com/5464020

In my ebook Is Your Lifestyle Putting Your Heart At Risk? we discuss the six greatest risks to your heart and the lifestyle changes you can make to mitigate them.

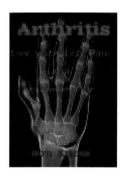

Arthritis – Live Wth Less Pain and Inflammation: Tips and Techniques You Can Use to Lessen the Pain and Inflammation

https://www.createspace.com/5457441

Discover Simple Tips & Information That Will Help Reduce The Painful Symptoms Of Arthritis!

You learn things like:
• Simple and effective information that will help you manage the pain and inflammation that comes along with arthritis, so that you can live an active, full life without debilitating pain.
• The different types of arthritis, their symptoms and how to alleviate their painful side effects.
• The pros and cons of over-the-counter arthritis medications, plus simple tips that will help you know how to choose the right supplements.

• Free, yet effective ways to get relief from arthritis pain and inflammation, so you don't have to suffer anymore. the effects arthritis can have significant impact on your physical and mental well-being, but this books shows you how to overcome its painful symptoms and live life relatively pain free.

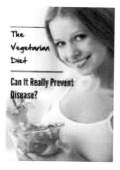

The Vegetarian Diet – Can It Really Prevent Disease?

https://www.createspace.com/5519874

Is a vegetarian diet right for you? Multiple studies have shown over and over that a vegetarian diet goes along way in preventing certain chronic diseases, such as:

• Heart Disease
• Cancer
• Diverticulitis
• Type 2 Diabetes
• Hypertension
• Obesity
• Kidney Failure

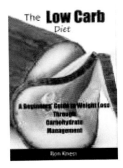

The Low Carb Diet: A Beginner's Guide to Weight Loss Through Carbohydrate Management

https://www.createspace.com/5416348

In my book "The Low-Carb Diet – A Beginners' Guide to Weight Loss Through Carbohydrate Management", I reveal a successful method of losing weight based in part on the amount and type of carbohydrates you consume.

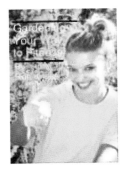

Gardening Your Way to Fitness: The Fun Way to Get Fit and Provide Beauty and Healthful Bounty for Your Family

https://www.createspace.com/5459564

The gym is a great place to stay fit during the colder seasons, but once the temperature turns warmer you want to spend more time outside. Plus, you'll have the benefit of fresh wholesome produce to enjoy by growing vegetables in your backyard garden.

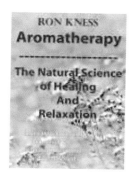

Aromatherapy - The Science of Healing and Relaxation: Learn How Essential Oils Elicit The Relaxation Response And Alter Mood

https://www.createspace.com/5714434

In my book Aromatherapy – The Science of Healing and Relaxation, we reveal the natural holistics methods you can use to heal the body from certain medical issues and to relive stress through relaxation. In particular we talk about:
• Aromatherapy - what it is and how it works
• Essential Oils – how the effects of certain aromas differs from others
• Recipes – how to make your own essential oil combinations

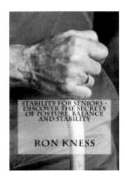

Stability for Seniors: Discover the Secrets of Posture, Balance and Stability

https://www.createspace.com/6096479

Many people sacrifice their health in pursuit of their career. They are so busy making a living that they neglect to make a life. The excuse that they do not have time to exercise is tossed about so frequently that they end up letting their health and fitness slide.

If you are not regularly active, you will have muscular atrophy over time. Your flexibility will decrease. Your core strength will diminish. As time progresses, you will be less limber and more rigid.

This is exactly how people age poorly. It's a process that has snowballed over time.

Only with regular exercise and a healthy diet can you have a body that is fit and has the ability to almost reverse aging.

If you have neglected your health for years and life seems to be a chore now because you can't get around without assistance, do not feel dejected.

You can remedy the situation. You can restore the strength, balance and stamina that you have lost. It is never too late to become what you might have been.

This guide will show you exactly what you need to do to restore your balance, strengthen your core and give you the ability to live life to its fullest. Read how …

About the Author

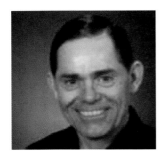 I grew up in Central Minnesota, where my parents own and operated a fishing resort. Once out of high school I tried a couple of semesters of college, only to quit halfway through the Spring term; I decided at that time that college wasn't for me.

Then I decided to follow my father's previous occupation as an auto mechanic. I graduated from a two-year of vocational training course and worked as a mechanic. While in vocational training, I decided to join the National Guard where I eventually ended up working full-time for 32 years.

So how does all of this relate to writing? In one of my leadership schools, the instructor, who was an English teacher at a juvenile detention center, presented writing to me in a whole new way - a way that started to develop my interest in working with words.

Fast forward about 40 years and I now have over 50 books listed on Amazon for Kindle and CreateSpace.

Besides my own writing, I also ghostwrite ebooks, reports, articles, blogs and do Kindle conversions for my clients on a variety of topics.

Today my wife and I live in Gold Canyon, AZ, where you'll find me happily sitting in my office typing away on my laptop as I work on my next book or ghostwriting project . . . that is if we are not traveling on a cruise ship - our new-found mode of travel.

If you like my book, please leave a review of it.

Printed in Great Britain
by Amazon